CANCER THE TREATMENT NO ONE BELIEVED

MY JOURNEY OF MIRACLES

I would like to extend my heartfelt gratitude to Dr. Hayden D. Henry and his wife, Lisa, for their unwavering generosity and boundless compassion. Your support and encouragement have been instrumental in bringing this book to life. Thank you for helping me share this journey and the miracle of discovering a power greater than ourselves, so others may find hope and inspiration.

Copyright © 2025, Earnest Best

Cancer The Treatment No One Believed:
My Journey of Miracles

ISBN: 979-8-218-58792-5

All rights reserved. No part of this publication may be reproduced, distributed, or transmitted in any form or by any means, including photocopying, recording, or other electronic or mechanical methods, without the prior written permission of the author, except in the case of brief quotations embodied in critical reviews and certain other noncommercial uses permitted by copyright law.

Book cover design and interior layout provided by Self Publish Me—Publishing Consulting and Book Design Services for Independent Authors, Oklahoma City, Oklahoma. Visit us at: www.selfpublishme.com, or email us at: info@selfpublishme.com

To Jack and Shirley McGee
and everyone battling cancer.

CANCER THE TREATMENT NO ONE BELIEVED

MY JOURNEY OF MIRACLES

Earnest Best

Edited by
Karen Sue Redlack

Dog Dewormer Put My Cancer in Remission With the Drug *FENBENDAZOLE* in it!

My name is Earnest Best. I have a friend who took a video of me about my cancer story and posted it on TikTok. It has gone out all over the world with over 50 million views and counting. It has been shared to Twitter (X), Facebook and Instagram. I don't know how far it has made it across the web. I also did a podcast with Dr. Karlfeldt, of Integrative Cancer Solutions, which can be found on my Facebook page. That podcast has been available worldwide. In response to all the media attention I have been contacted by a great number of people asking me about using the dog dewormer that has the drug Fenbendazole in it to treat my cancer. I have been asked to share my story, the protocol, and follow up. I have been in remission from cancer for three years as of December 2024. I have received no treatments or surgeries other than to remove the tumor from my bladder, to have a biopsy done, to see if it was cancer.

I'm not a doctor or affiliated with any medical platforms. I'm not promoting the sale of any one product, story, or the sale of anyone's goods. I'm a 63-year-old pipe liner who came down with an incurable form of highly aggressive cancer, Plasmacytoid Urothelial Carcinoma, that appeared in my bladder in December of 2021. I went to the restroom one morning upon waking up for work in Eunice, New Mexico, just south of Hobbs, New Mexico. I was a Heavy Equipment Operator, running a 1055 Vermeer Trencher, digging ditches for the construction of new pipelines. I leaned over to flush the toilet and noticed the urine I passed looked like pure tomato juice (it was blood). I immediately became very concerned. Later that morning, before leaving for work, I used the restroom again and used a container to catch the urine to get a closer look at it. As I was trying to urinate, the flow stopped and I couldn't complete it. Suddenly, a huge blood clot came out. I took a photo of it and saved it.

I went to work and informed my boss about what was going on, still passing blood throughout the day. My boss told me I needed to go see a doctor. After work that day, I was out in west Texas and New Mexico. I went to Odessa, Texas to the emergency room (ER) there. When I arrived, I told them what was going on and showed them the photos. I was placed in a room. The doctor came in and I showed him the photos. He ordered a urine sample and a CT-Scan, along with an EKG, to see what was going on. After quite a wait he came in with the results. He said, "Mr. Best it doesn't look good. It appears that you have some tumors in your bladder that might be cancer. And your heart is enlarged, along with an irregular heartbeat." He told me I needed to follow up with a urologist as soon as possible (ASAP) to get the tumors checked out. I left and returned to Eunice, New Mexico. This is the point where my thoughts started going crazy. I believe the mind is the battlefield. Our thoughts can lead us to destruction or recovery. The mind and body are powerful.

I went to work the following day and told my boss the outcome of my medical visits. I began making phone calls to find a local urologist who could see me ASAP. I found one in Lovington, New Mexico, just North of Hobbs. They made an appointment for me on January 12, 2022. I went in for the appointment and showed them the medical records they had given me in Odessa, Texas. After they reviewed them, along with the CD's included, they came in to talk to me and check me out. He said if I had the time that day, he wanted to go up into my bladder with a camera to see what was there. I agreed and he did. I was able to photograph the tumors he found. He said they were about the size of big grapes. He needed to take them out to get a pathologist report, to see if they were cancerous or not. After reviewing the records and EKG, as well as noticing all the fluid I had in my legs, he wanted me to see the cardiologist at that clinic. He needed to know if the cardiologist thought I would be able to undergo the surgery to remove the tumors. His nurse took me down to the cardiologist's office to schedule an appointment to come back in and follow up with him. I came back and he ordered many tests and procedures. After several days and many appointments he went over his findings. They found that I needed to be placed on oxygen because my level was in the 70's. He ordered oxygen for me. He said I was in bad shape with severe heart problems and that my CO_2 levels were too high. He wasn't going to allow the urologist to perform the surgery at that small clinic because they wouldn't be able to save me if something unforeseen were to happen. He sent me to University Hospital in Albuquerque, New Mexico to see the urologist and a heart surgeon. They called and set up an appointment in February 2022. I drove myself there and went to see the urologist first. She received all my records from Lovington and sent me to see the heart surgeon right away. He came in, checked me out and admitted me that day. He said I was in bad shape. They went right to work performing multiple scans, tests and procedures. They worked on me for nine days. He came in to tell me the results after seven days. I had Congestive Heart Failure, Severe Pulmonary Hypertension, Chronic Hypoxic Respiratory Failure, Afib and Sleep Apnea, the sleep study showed I was bad enough to need a Bi-PAP machine. They started me on a lot of different meds and got me stable enough, so they thought, to undergo the surgery to remove the tumors.

The mental torture was the worst part of all of this. The thoughts about maybe having cancer and now all this heart stuff and the oxygen issues were my battlefield. Thank God I had been involved in a twelve-step program of recovery from alcohol and drugs for many years. I had ten years clean and sober in April of 2022. I attended meetings and shared my condition with friends in the program. I had a great support group to help me deal with my mental anguish. Not once had any thoughts of relapse or the obsession to use ever come to me. My mind and thoughts began what I believe is the worst part of getting this diagnosis, not knowing if I have cancer or if I was going to die. The thoughts of regret for the things I have been too caught up into life to enjoy, fears of the unknown. It was a world of endless thoughts and emotions.

The urologist scheduled my surgery for the last week of March 2022. I left and went home. I returned in March, checked in and was prepared for surgery. The thoughts of not being able to survive all this were enormous. I constantly prayed to God to help me accept whatever was about to happen. I asked God to protect my crazy mind, the thoughts that were running through my mind and all the emotions that were following this situation. It was scary because they told me that there was a 50-50 chance of something going wrong with my heart. And with the condition I was in, I wouldn't survive. I was given a possible death sentence that day and for the first time I was in a place I had never stood before. If you have ever been in this position you know what I say is true. I was somewhat afraid, but deep inside I felt like it was going to be okay either way. I knew it was in God's Hands and the hands of the surgeon performing the procedure. They took me in, put me under and performed the surgery, then I woke up in the Heart Ward.

As soon as I regained my awareness, I was grateful I woke up, but was confused as to why I was there. They told me they were having problems getting my oxygen level up and that during the surgery they had some problems. Because I was so overweight, they weren't able to push down as hard as they needed to, and they couldn't remove all of the tumor that was in the throat of my bladder. It turned out to be the one that was cancerous. In response to my oxygen levels, I informed them that in my drinking and drugging days I liked to fight. My nose had been broken a few times and I wasn't able to breathe through it, so I pulled the hose from my nose and put it in my mouth. My oxygen began to rise right away. The doctors laughed and said, "WOW that's good to know. We will have to add that question to our procedures." After that, they brought in a full face mask for me to use to keep my oxygen level up.

They informed me that they were able to get one tumor out completely, but the other one was in the throat of my bladder and was about a 5.5. I asked what that meant and the doctor said about the size of a lemon. So the tumors had grown from a big grape to a lemon in three months. He then said that they weren't able to get it all out and had to leave part of it in me. Because of the problems they were having with me they had to stop the surgery before they could remove the tumors completely. I was told I would get the pathologist's report in a couple of days and we would see if it was cancerous or not. I was told I would go home in a few days with the catheter in. They came in to give me the pathologist's results and said, "Mr. Best it doesn't look good. One tumor was benign, the one in the throat of your bladder was positive for cancer. It is a highly aggressive, rare type called Plasmacytoid Urothelial Carcinoma. The report said:

Plasmacytoid (Positive CD 138)

Grade: HIGH

Microscopic extent of the tumor: Invades into the Lamina

Pathological Stage: PT 1

Tumor cells are positive for CK 7 and CD 138

She then went on to explain the one good thing is that it's at an early stage one. And as of now, it was into the wall of my bladder and the lamina. The lamina is a thin layer of connective tissue that surrounds the urothelium. It contains blood vessels, nerves and glands. The cancer hadn't broken into the muscle and spread out YET. She explained this type of rare cancer doesn't respond to chemo or radiation treatments. There were no known treatments that worked. The only other option was radical surgery to remove my bladder, prostate, lymph nodes and put a bag on my side to collect the urine. Due to my condition, I was inoperable. She was sorry there wasn't anything they could do. I then asked how long I had and she said, "That is between you and God, maybe six months to a year." They didn't know how aggressive the cancer was going to be since it was disturbed and they weren't able to remove it all. I was overwhelmed and felt fear and depression for a few moments. My mind began the battle telling me, "It's over Earnest." I made it out alive from the surgery (THANK GOD) and now another DEATH SENTENCE! This one sounded more serious!

I had a friend who came to get me and bring me back to Eunice, New Mexico, where I was living at that time, with the catheter still in. I called and scheduled an appointment with the first urologist in Lovington to have him remove it after about ten days. I spoke with his nurse, told her all that had happened, and asked her if they could get the records from the hospital so he could review them and give me a second opinion. I went to see him and he removed the catheter. He sat down and began telling me the same thing the urologist in Albuquerque told me about the reports. I asked him how long I might have and he said the same thing, "Mr. Best no one can tell you. That's between you and God, but it doesn't look good."

I left feeling overwhelmed with emotions. For the first time in many years the thought to drink and get high entered my mind from somewhere. Thank God the 12 step program I was in taught me that the obsession to drink is where the problem begins. I'm powerless over these thoughts entering my mind, but God can help me fight them off if I will turn my thinking and emotions over to Him each day. I have learned that in order to recover I must pray and meditate every morning, surrendering my mind, thoughts and emotions over to Him. Asking Him to put a hedge of protection around them all and to direct my thinking and path each day, asking Him for the right thoughts and actions to win the battlefield of my mind. They taught me that no human power could stop those thoughts from coming into my mind and no human power could stop me from listening to those thoughts that turn into an obsession. It had happened many times in the past and I was truly powerless over them. I came to believe that what they had said was indeed true. I relapsed many times because I was powerless at the moment those thoughts would come. But because this time in recovery I followed the directions of a man who had been through this and found the solution. I worked on my spiritual malady. I found a relationship with the only power that could help me and put the next right thoughts in my mind. Believe me, the battle was on! But He was right there to help me. Right after the thoughts of relapse came, the next thought was to try to give myself over for research to try to maybe find a cure for this type of highly aggressive incurable cancer! I wanted to try to save others from this disease.

I called MD Anderson and they told me that they couldn't help me. I called another one in Arizona and was told the same thing. I thought, "Well, what now?" So, I decided to post on Facebook what was going on with me and let my friends and family know about all this. That's when it all started. A friend and former girlfriend from 40 years ago, Retha McBroom, texted me and told me she had a friend who had cancer and was supposed to die. She took some kind of dog dewormer that had treated her cancer, was still alive and cancer free. I asked her what kind of dog dewormer was used. She didn't know, but would try to find out. Then another friend, Diana Litton, who works as a nurse in Oklahoma City texted me and told me she works with a lady who had ovarian cancer and was supposed to die, but started taking a dog dewormer that had treated her as well. Then another text from David Jones, an old boss. He said his preacher from a Cowboy Church in Fairfield, Texas wanted to talk to me if I didn't mind, I thought he wanted to make sure I was right with God and ready to die. So, I told him sure, have him call me. He did a few days later and told me that he had a couple of women in his church who had cancer and had both taken some kind of dog dewormer that had treated their cancer. The treatment saved their lives and they were cancer free. I again asked what kind, but he didn't know either and would try to find out. I hadn't talked to these people in person to ask so I called on my best friend "GOOGLE" to help me. I Googled, "Dog Dewormer that kills Cancer" and sure enough something popped up, "Dog Dewormer" with the drug FENBENDAZOLE in it. A story about a man named Joe Tippen from Edmond, Oklahoma. who had a veterinarian tell him about the drug Fenbendazole possibly killing cancer also popped up. His story can be found on Facebook and YouTube. I started doing a world of research and found many others who had used the drug Fenbendazole and were found to have no evidence of disease (NED).

So here I am facing a "Death Sentence" from this cancer that has no known cure and people are telling me about a possible treatment. Right away my thoughts and mind became the battlefield. I told myself, "I'm not taking no dog dewormer!" I began to read about the side effects and found nothing at that time. Then the thought came to me, "What have you got to lose Earnest, you're going to die anyway?" I laughed at that thought and drove into Hobbs to the Tractor Supply and asked where to find the dog dewormer. The young lady volunteered to take me back and show me where it was and help me. She said, "You are supposed to use the pet's weight as a guide to give it to them." She wanted to know how much my pet weighed, so I laughed, looked down at myself and said, "Oh about 350." She responded with, "MY GOD, WHAT KIND OF DOG DO YOU HAVE?" I laughed again and told her about my research and having cancer and that I was supposed to be going to die soon. She then said that I wouldn't believe there had been a few others who came in looking for this and had also used it to treat their cancer. I believed that here again the Spirit of the Universe was putting others in my pathway to give me the directions to treat me and save my life, which indeed, it has done so far to date.

I read where Joe Tippen had taken 222 mg doses each day along with other stuff he took as well which I found on his podcast and profile on the Internet. As I was doing my research, I discovered that the dog dewormer in the blue box had three, two-gram packets, in each packet there was 222 mg/g per gram. So that told me that a two-gram packet had a total of 444 mgs of Fenbendazole in them. A gram has 1000 mgs in them. So 778 mgs is a buffer and other things. Since there wasn't any way to separate the Fenbendazole from the other stuff, I could try to take just 222 mgs of Fenbendazole, which is what his protocol said. I simplified it, not trying to divide the packet because who knows which half has the Fenbendazole in it or how much. I read so much craziness online and people telling people to do crazy things like that, I decided to double his dose. I had active cancer that had been disturbed in surgery and part of the cancerous tumor was left in my bladder. I wanted to try to kill the cancer ASAP, so each two-gram packet I took had a total of 2000 mgs in them with a total of 444 mgs of that 2000 mgs was Fenbendazole. I wanted to hit it hard like taking antibiotics for a bad infection. I read where Fenbendazole doesn't dissolve in water, so I poured the first dose in a little water to see what happened. And sure enough, just part of the packet dissolved and turned the water white. And on the top of the water was what appeared to be the Fenbendazole. Some had sunk to the bottom, but didn't in fact dissolve, so I ate breakfast and drank it to start the journey of being cancer free. This was the first part of May in 2022.

My research into cancer taught me a lot I didn't know. The research into Fenbendazole taught me about the drug and its effect on cancer cells and parasites in humans, as well as all the diseases and things they do to us humans. My research really opened up a whole new world of insight and learning.

I decided that I would put the whole packet into Applesauce after that or just mix it with food. The research told me it needed to have some kind of fat or oil to dissolve in so the body could process it better. I then decided that since I had this type of cancer, I would take it twice a day to hit it hard to try to kill the tumor and the cancer, and so it did! I did one whole two-gram packet in the morning and one two-gram packet at night with my meals. That was a total of 888 mgs of Fenbendazole each day along with 500 mgs of turmeric/curcumin and 500 mgs of magnesium once a day.

I spent weeks studying about cancer, parasites, food we eat, the chemicals we are exposed to daily, how to kill cancer, food to eat to help kill it, food and water not to drink, herbs to take and natural remedies to take to kill cancer and parasites. It would take volumes of books to write down all of what I have learned. I encourage each person who reads this to start your research, look things up and find the knowledge you need to fight this fight. The first and foremost thing that I suggest is to fight the battle of the mind! Thoughts come from some place beyond our consciousness. A thought just comes and enters our minds. For me, I believe this is what's called the Spiritual Realm. I have experienced that I can't stop negative thoughts from coming into my mind. I had thoughts of trying to control my negative thoughts only to fail time and time again.

When they told me I had this incurable, highly aggressive, cancer that was going to kill me, that they couldn't help me, the crazy thoughts began for a short time. Feelings of fear, depression, anxiety, guilt, fear of the unknown, fear of going to Hell if it really exists. In the first 30 minutes I had a ton of thoughts, emotions and ideas. It was crazy to say the least. Unless you have experienced it, then it's hard to relate. But for those who have, you know what I say is true!!

On April 21, 2022 I was given the pathologist report in Albuquerque, New Mexico that confirmed I was positive for Plasmacytoid Carcinoma Cancer with a death sentence attached. It's been over two years now and I'm still cancer free today. I still take 222 mgs of Fenbendazole. I take it for a week out of every month as a follow up along with turmeric/curcumin and magnesium.

MY PROTOCOL TO START

Dog dewormer, two-gram packet (444 Mgs of Fenbendazole)

Twice a day (7 days a week) with my meal. (blue box)

500 mg pill of Turmeric/Curcumin (once a day 7 days a week)

500mg pill of Magnesium (once a day 7 days a week)

I read where cancer and parasites feed off glucose (sugar). So I stopped all sugar intake, sodas, candy, any kind of sweets, and any other kind of glucose intake. I started eating all kinds of fruits Blueberries, Strawberries, Avocados, Citrus fruits, Bananas (a lot of the fruits have a natural sweetness in them). I ate a lot of Oatmeal, Eggs, Fish, Turkey, Chicken, Beans of all kinds, Beets and many other foods. I found out that the processed meats, red meat, pork and just a whole world of things I was eating wasn't good for me. I had no Idea that food was such a big contributor to causing cancer, along with all the chemicals and preservatives that are put in our food.

By this time, it was the first part of May 2022. I told my boss I didn't know if this dog dewormer was going to work and save my life or not, but I needed to quit my job. I had to return home to get my affairs in order and prepare to die. I have family members who died from cancer and it's not a pretty site. I put in my two-week notice and worked through it. Then I quit and returned to Ardmore, Oklahoma. I came to a longtime friend's house and rented a room from him. He said he would be there to walk through all this with me and help me in any way he could. I was still taking my protocol, the same way, not knowing if it was working or not. The bleeding from the surgery had just about stopped. I was still using a container when I used the restroom. On Memorial Day, May 30, 2022, something strange happened. I was collecting my urine in a container to check for blood or tissue of any kind. By this time my urine had started to clear up with only a few drops of blood and white particles. But that morning I was using the restroom and all of a sudden, my urine flow stopped, I tried to go some more, but nothing would come out. I didn't know what was going on. I remembered when I was a kid and my cousin and I would be down on the river camping and fishing with my Grandpa and Dad and we sometimes would see who could urinate the furthest. So I did the process to pressure up and when I released it, I was amazed at what came out into the container. A bunch of tissue looking like fat trimmed off of a steak, about a big tablespoon full, along with some blood. I was shocked. I collected it and saved it to photograph it. I put it in alcohol to try to preserve it so I could show it to the doctors. (I have the photos. The doctor kept the tissue.)

I contacted the Oklahoma University (OU) Cancer Center in Oklahoma City. The urologist in Lovington, New Mexico had been trying to help me find some place that I might be able to get some help. He contacted me and said they would see me. I had an appointment to meet with the leading physician there in July 2022. I brought all my medical records, CD's, from the cardiologist, urologist, the pathologist's report and everything I had collected. I went in for my first visit and they ordered me to have CT-Scans done, with and without enhancement, to see what was going on with the cancer and the tumor that had been left in my bladder. I came back, had all the scans, waited around for a few hours and returned to see the doctor to go over the results. I brought the jar with the tissue in it I had passed to show him. I wanted to see if he could tell me what it was. I hadn't told any of them about taking the dog dewormer yet. I read that Fenbendazole hadn't had any medical research done or received any approval by the Center for Disease Control (CDC), or any medical field of study. So I kept it to myself. The only doctor I confided in was the urologist in New Mexico about me taking it prior to returning to Oklahoma.

I waited for the doctor to come in and I decided that I would record his conversation with me when he came in (which I have today). When he came into the room his first words were, "Mr. Best I have some bits of good news, I don't see anything on any of the scans, no signs of cancer or even the tumor that they said they left in your bladder. What kind of treatments have you had?" I was shocked! I told him what they had told me in Albuquerque about this type of cancer. I told him they had no treatments available that worked because it didn't respond to chemo or radiation. There wasn't anything they could do for me and I was inoperable due to all of my heart problems. The bottom line was that I might have six months to one year to live. I asked him if he had reviewed the pathologist slides from New Mexico to see if it was indeed this rare and highly aggressive type of Plasmacytoid Carcinoma Cancer. He stated that he had and also had the pathologist there at OU Cancer Center review them. Both agreed that it was indeed the rare and aggressive Plasmacytoid Carcinoma Cancer. I then asked him, "So you don't see any signs of cancer or the tumor they left in my bladder?" He said, "No sir, not from what I can tell." I said, "Praise God!" I told him about taking the dog dewormer with Fenbendazole in it and that I had passed all that stuff on Memorial Day. I pulled the jar from my bag and showed it to him, asking him if it might be the tumor they had left. His response was, "It looks like it might be, but since you put it in alcohol I wouldn't be able to get a pathologist report to confirm it. But it possibly could be. You need to see a urologist to have a procedure done again to go up into your bladder to get a visual to make sure." I know longer have the jar. He kept it, but I do have a photo of it. He went on to say that the dog dewormer was a parasitic drug and that it had no research done in the field of cancer. I asked him again "SO YOU DON'T SEE NO CANCER OR THE TUMOR?" He said again, "NO SIR,

NOT FROM WHAT I COULD SEE." I again said, "THANK YOU GOD!"

He then went on to tell me that the only way to make sure that all the Cancer was dead or gone was to remove my bladder, prostate and lymph nodes to keep it from coming back a few years down the road, and that he would put a bag on my side to catch my urine. He said the worst-case scenario would be we do the surgery and send off my bladder for a pathologist report and if it comes back negative, all the cancer cells were dead. He said it was up to me. I told him to give me a few days to decide, but to go ahead and set it up and I would let him know.

This was the first proof that I had that the dog dewormer with Fenbendazole in it was indeed working and had performed a miracle! It appeared I was NED! I was amazed that he wanted to do the surgery because the doctors in New Mexico said I wasn't in any shape to undergo the radical type of surgery to do all that because of my heart and lung condition. When I reminded him of what they had told me, he asked about the medical records from them. I told him I had given them all copies of all that documentation. Then I wondered if he had even read any of the reports and records I had given them because if he had he would have known all this. I told him I would let him know my decision and I left with all this recorded on my phone.

At that time, I was on oxygen 24/7. In New Mexico, they told me I had invasive high grade Plasmacytoid cancer, non-operable to remove the bladder and it was resistant to chemotherapy and radiation, Congestive Heart Failure, Severe Pulmonary Hypertension, on high doses of diuretics, Chronic Hypoxic respiratory failure requiring oxygen 24/7 and I was pre-diabetic. He knew none of this, all of which was in the records I had given them.

I know this is a lot to read about. But what I want to share with whomever reads this is that no matter what storms of life come at us, there is always a flicker of HOPE!! If we just believe, that makes miracles possible.

My life so far has been an awesome journey with so much to share. My journey with cancer, heart problems, alcoholism and drug addiction, recovery from those addictions, depression, failed suicide attempts, abandonments, foster homes, many deaths of loved ones, prison for five and one-half years on a 15 to Life sentence for drugs, because of the decisions I made, failed relationships, a divorce, death of my stepson and so many other things. The list could go on and on. I know all of us have a story we could tell. Running through people's lives like a hurricane, leaving the disaster behind only to move on to another town or state, blaming others to justify my actions, not knowing all along it was something within me. BUT WHAT? That's the age-old riddle! I thank God every day for Him not giving up on me, that He has kept me alive and saved me from a lot. I thank God, He has helped me lay aside all the old ideas I had about religion, about old beliefs, some unrealistic and some delusional, some wrong and completely off track.

I had the video I recorded when the cancer doctor came in to give me the results from the CT scans. I wanted to let some of my family and friends listen to it and try to get some help from them to make a decision on what I should do. I left the hospital and went to see my stepsister, Karion Dalton Goff, (who we call Sudy) to let her listen to the recording and give me her advice. She, too, has been in the same program of recovery as I for over 20 years. I have experienced that we can get Spiritual Guidance through others if we seek it. On the way to see Sudy I did a lot of praying thanking God for putting all those people in my life to tell me about the dog dewormer with Fenbendazole to kill my cancer and thanked Him for putting that veterinarian in Joe Tippens life, telling him about Fenbendazole and saving his life. On the way I had lots of things going on in my mind. I thought, "WOW! THIS DOG DEWORMER HAS REALLY DONE THE IMPOSSIBLE. IT HAS TAKEN AWAY MY CANCER." I remember thinking why on earth would I do this procedure and go through all that if I DON'T HAVE CANCER TODAY! I thought that would be like pulling my teeth before I got a cavity. The next thought I recall was maybe spiritual in nature, it was, "JUST HAVE FAITH EARNEST. I GOT THIS," accompanied with goose bumps! When I arrived at Sudy's work I went in and sat down, told her what was going on and let her listen to the recording. Not telling her that I was there to seek out her spiritual guidance. She listened and afterwards responded with, "That's crazy. Why on earth go through all that if he sees no cancer or tumors?" When she said that the same thought popped into my mind again, "HAVE FAITH EARNEST I GOT THIS." So after a short visit, I left for Ardmore, praying while thanking God for everything.

When I arrived back home, I went to see a few other friends that I felt could give me some spiritual direction and help me make up my mind on what I should do.

They all told me the same thing. So my mind was made up. I was going to have faith that all was going as it should. I called the cancer center and told the doctor's office I wasn't going to have the surgery. This all happened around July 15, 2022. I was still following my protocol that I had been taking. This was about two and one half months I had been on the Dog Dewormer, taking two packets a day, for a total of 888 mgs of Fenbendazole, along with the other stuff. It appeared from the CT scans that I was cancer free.

This journey since December 2021, in the ER at Odessa, Texas, when the cancerous tumors were found until July 2022, eight months later, has been one of the most amazing spiritual journeys I have ever been on. From having a DEATH SENTENCE handed to me to having a MIRACLE happen and being CANCER FREE without ever having any kind of treatments or surgeries done, other than the surgery to try to remove the tumors from my bladder. Had it not been for the cancer, I never would have known about the major heart blockage or my widowmaker that was a ticking time bomb waiting to kill me!

I went to see my primary care doctor and for the first time shared all this with him. Telling him about the cancer and the protocol, showing him all the records I had and letting him listen to the recordings I acquired along the way from OU Cancer Center. He stated that he heard something about this dog dewormer and cancer, but that there hadn't been any medical research into it. But he was curious since I had shown him all the stuff I had and proof up to this point. He asked me if I would be willing to work with him and do some more research and tests to see if it was really working. I said, "Of course, let's do this." He ordered a full PET Scan along with an MRI of my brain, and more blood work. The PET Scan and MRI were both done on February 7, 2023. A few days after the scans I returned to get the results and visit with him. All the tests came back NED, no signs of cancer or tumors anywhere! He stated, off the record, that since our visit he had started doing his own research. He found out that the medical field had indeed known about Fenbendazole killing cancer for a while now, but wasn't letting it out. He said he was upset because he had lost family members, along with many patients to cancer, that might have been able to live had he known. So here is another one that's finding out about Fenbendazole and here I am in person with all the records, recordings, scans, PET Scan, MRI, and living proof that this stuff works as I am CANCER FREE! He wanted me to go see a urologist next to have a procedure done where they go up into my bladder with a camera to look around and see if the cancer might be trying to come back. This was the same procedure that they had done in Lovington, New Mexico when they found the tumors. So he sent me and I went. The procedure went well. Since I was awake, I was able to videotape it all, which I have on my phone. The procedure results came back all clear, showing nothing but scar tissue from where the tumors were and no sign of anything left behind from the removal of them. The tissue I passed and collected had to have been the tumor that was left behind in New Mexico. The tumor had died and came out. "PRAISE GOD AGAIN."

My primary care doctor sent me to see the cancer doctor in Ardmore to get with them to see what they could find. I went and saw them. They ordered blood work, reviewed all my records and asked me what kind of treatments I had. I told them NONE. He said, "But you had a Plasmacytoid Carcinoma." I said, "Yes." He then asked about the surgery to remove my bladder and I said, "They didn't do the procedure." He then said, "Mr. Best, I don't see anything in all the tests, scans, blood work or anything that shows any cancer or tumors. What have you done?" So, I told him! I shared with him my journey with the dog dewormer with Fenbendazole in it and I told him about some of my research along with the story about Joe Tippen. I showed him the photos I had on my phone and he didn't seem to like that too much. He said since I refused the surgery to remove my bladder and other stuff that the only option was to keep seeing the urologist to monitor what's going on, do blood tests to keep an eye on my progress and to keep doing whatever I had been doing. So, I got up and left.

Today is August 19, 2024, as I write this. It's been a crazy journey for sure. It's been over two and one half years since the first scans that showed possible cancer tumors and passing all the blood. As of today, I'm still cancer free.

EVERYTHING had shown me to be NED. I thought I would try to see what Joe Tippens follow up protocol was as he was cancer free as well. I decided to try to find just Fenbendazole pills to take and I found them on Amazon from a company called Snare Lab. Since I had been taking 888 mgs a day, I decided to cut it in half for a while and drop back to 444 mgs a day. So I ordered 444 mgs pills, a 90 count bottle, from Amazon. They cost $109.00. I started taking them as soon as they arrived. I left everything else the same in my protocol. I was only taking one pill of Fenbendazole a day. I did this for several months then decided to give my body a break. I ordered 222 mgs from Fenben lab because they were out of the Snare Lab brand. I then decided to take 1 222 mg pill for one week out of each month and that's what I do today.

My aftercare protocol is as follows:

1 222 mg pill of Fenbendazole, once a day, for one week a month

1 500 mg turmeric/curcumin once a day

1 500 mg magnesium once a day

1 multivitamin once a day

These are some of the photos I have taken during this journey. I have all the other documents and records to prove my journey with cancer and show to anyone upon request.

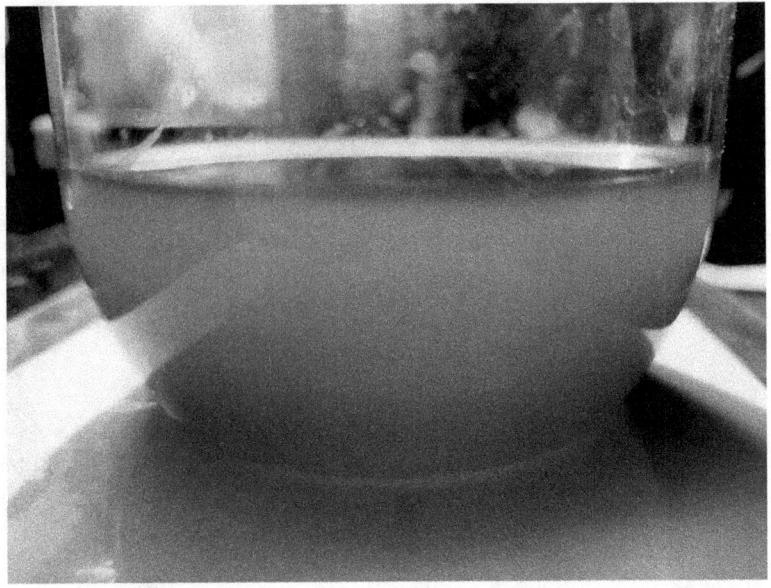

The blood I passed the first morning in my urine

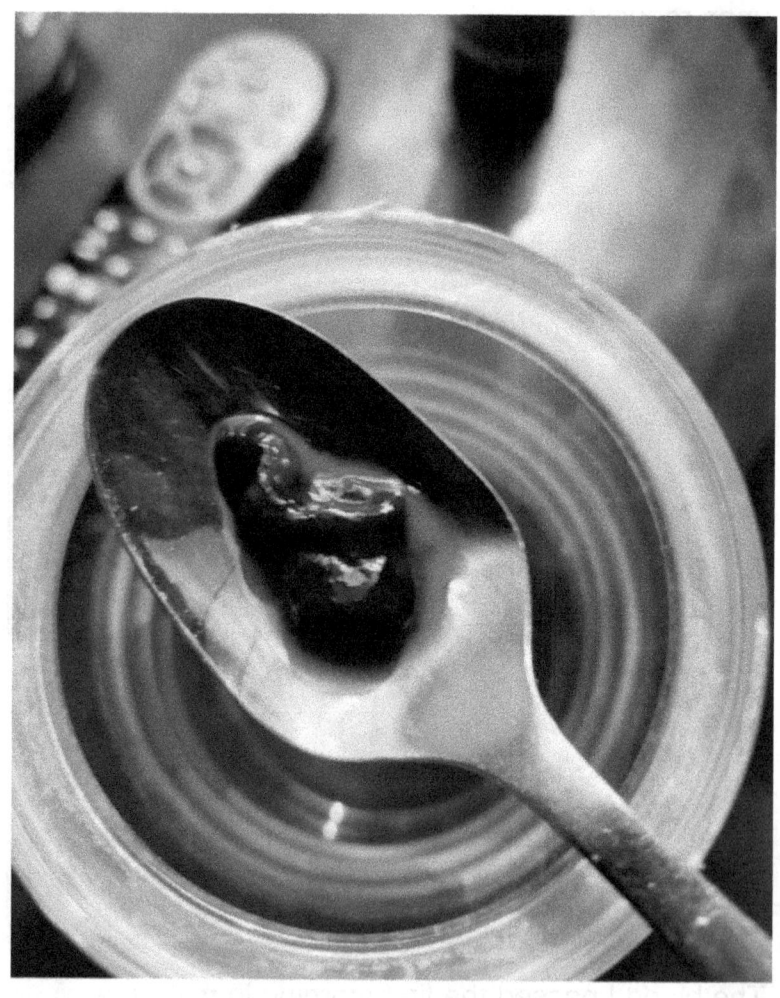
Blood clot I passed.

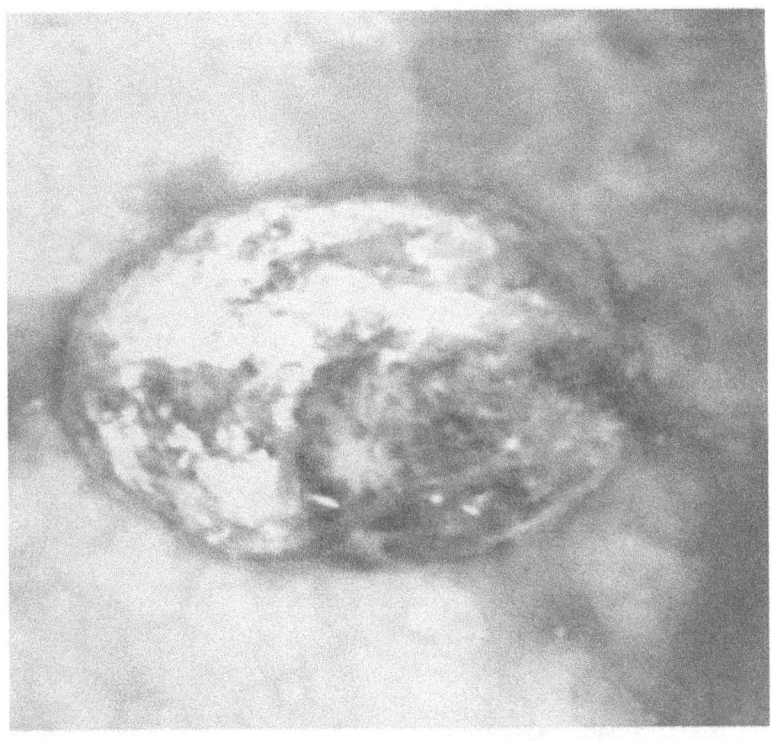

One of the tumors the urologist found in my bladder.

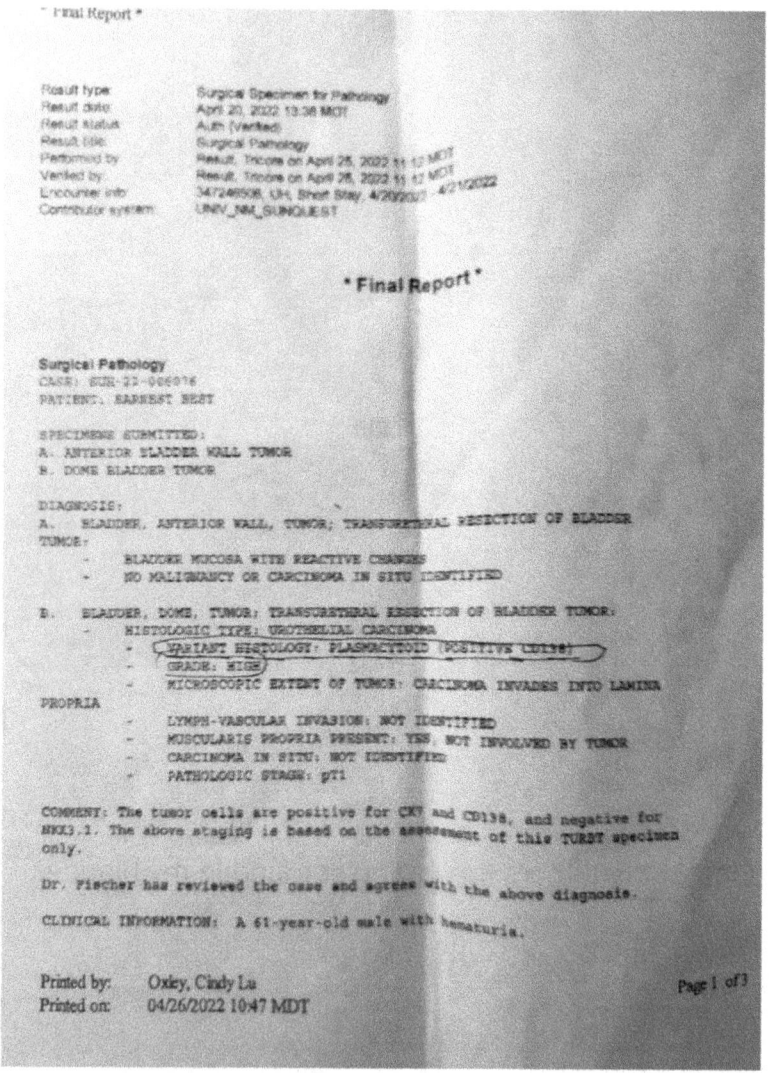

Pathologist's report of the tumors.

Pathologist's report of the tumors.

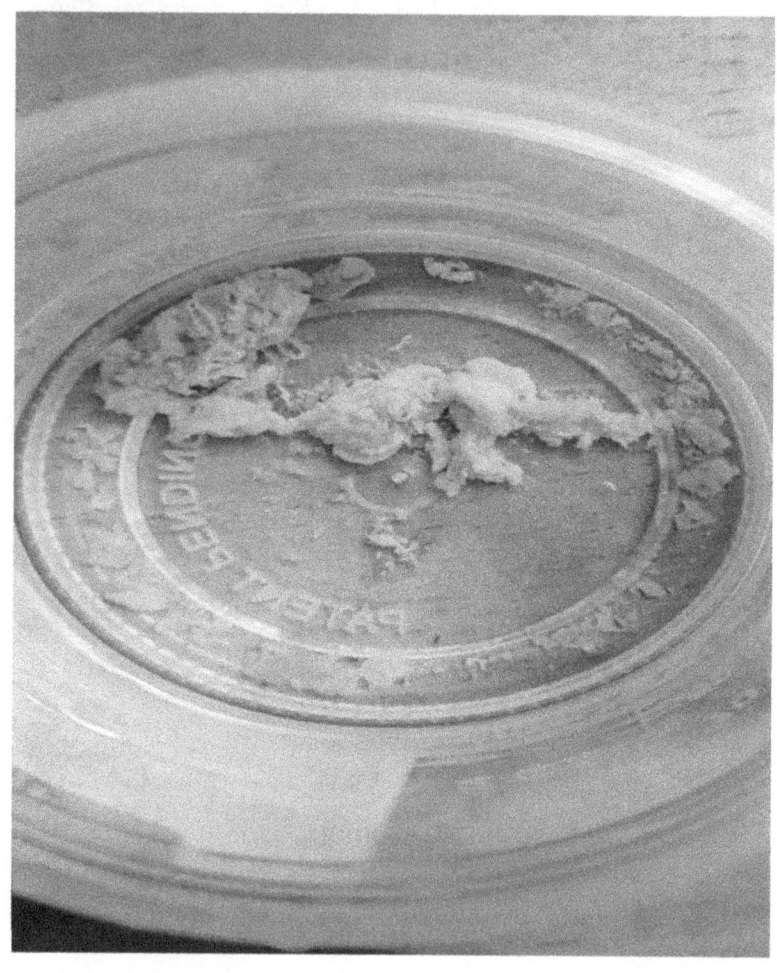

Tumor I had on Memorial Day. It changed color after I put it in alcohol. It was pinkish, yellow, red.
Like trimmings from a steak.

LOVINGTON MEDICAL CLINIC PRIMARY CARE
1600 N MAIN ST STE A
LOVINGTON NM 88260-2830
Phone: 575-396-6611
Fax: 575-396-9068

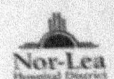

May 5, 2022

RE:
Patient: **Earnest Best**
Date of Birth: **1/16/1961**
Date of Visit: **4/28/2022**

To Whom It May Concern:

The purpose of this letter is to document significant chronic health conditions that impair activities of daily living for Earnest Best. I have been Mr. Best's primary care physician over the past year since his diagnosis of bladder cancer.

Earnest Best's health issues and their affect on employment meet the definition of disability.

Significant health impairments
Renal system
    Invasive, high-grade carcinoma of the bladder- Managed by urology [Dr Montgomery]. Nonoperable and resistant to chemotherapy. Patient requires extensive appointments with specialists, underwent recent resection requiring catheterization, frequent bathroom access limiting ability to perform any and all required tasks for employment.
Cardiovascular system.
    Congestive heart failure, Sever pulmonary hypertension- Managed by UNM cardiology [Dr. Andre] in Albuquerque, New Mexico. High-dose daily diuretics required. Monitoring of water intake, daily weights, and frequent bathroom usage but severe notations on patient's ability to maintain employment.
Respiratory system:
    Chronic hypoxic respiratory failure- Requires 24/7 supplemental oxygenation.
Endocrine system:
    Prediabetes- Patient requires frequent monitoring of blood glucose as well as attendance of diabetes education.

If you have any questions or concerns, please don't hesitate to call.

Sincerely,

Seth Coombs, MD

Primary care doctors letter in New Mexico.

CANCER THE TREATMENT NO ONE BELIEVED *MY JOURNEY OF MIRACLES*

```
EXAMS:                                              CPT:
007315028 CT ABD AND PELV W-WO CONTRAST             74178
```

CT ABDOMEN AND PELVIS WITH AND WITHOUT CONTRAST DATED 7/15/2022 9:19 AM

HISTORY: Bladder cancer

COMPARISON: None

TECHNIQUE: Helical tomographic images of the abdomen pelvis are obtained before and after the uncomplicated intravenous injection of 120 cc Isovue-370 utilizing a CT urographic protocol. Multiple sagittal and coronal reformatted images are provided for review. Total exam DLP = 4220 mGy-cm.

FINDINGS:

Imaged lung bases demonstrate no focal consolidation or pulmonary mass. Imaged heart is not enlarged. There is no demonstrated pleural nor pericardial effusion.

The liver demonstrates a smooth contour, without suspicious enhancing liver lesion. The spleen is not enlarged. There is no pancreatic ductal dilatation. Gallbladder is present without radiopaque intraluminal stone. No intrahepatic or extrahepatic biliary ductal dilatation.

Bilateral adrenal glands demonstrate no focal mass. Bilateral kidneys demonstrate symmetric contrast enhancement. No hydronephrosis or perinephric fluid collection. No demonstrated nephrolithiasis or enhancing renal mass. Ureters are decompressed. Urinary bladder is distended without intraluminal stone or focal wall abnormality. Prostate and bilateral seminal vesicles demonstrate no acute process.

Gastrointestinal tract demonstrate no evidence of bowel obstruction. There is no evidence of free intraperitoneal air or free fluid. Sigmoid colon diverticulosis is seen without CT evidence of acute diverticulitis. There is no evidence of free intraperitoneal air or free fluid.

Abdominal aorta is of normal caliber with diffuse Atherosclerotic calcification. Celiac axis, superior mesenteric artery, bilateral renal arteries, and inferior mesenteric artery are all grossly patent at their origins. Hepatic veins and portal venous system appear grossly patent.

```
PAGE  1                     Signed Report                    (CONTINUED)
                     OU MEDICAL CENTER - OU PHYSICIANS BUILDING
825 N.E. 10th                    CT SCAN                 PHONE: (405) 271-1654
Oklahoma City, OK 73104     CONSULTATION REPORT          FAX:   (405) 271-1977
-----------------------------------------------------------------------------
LOC/RM: EA.CT/              PACS ID: E1042370           MRN:      E900002082
PT. TYPE: REG CLI           CAMPUS: AU        PT:               BEST,EARNEST
ACCT#: E00679567148                           DOB: 01/16/1961 AGE: 61   SEX: M
-----------------------------------------------------------------------------
ORD PROV: 1891954095 Cross,Brian Wesley  MD    EXAM START: 07/15/22 0919
ATT PROV: 1891954095 Cross,Brian Wesley  MD    EXAM ENDED: 07/15/22 0919
ADMISSION CLINICAL DATA: C67.9 MALIGNANT NEOPLASM OF BLADDER, UNS
```

```
EXAMS:                                              CPT:
007315028 CT ABD AND PELV W-WO CONTRAST             74178
```

The surrounding soft tissues demonstrate no acute abnormality. Osseous structures demonstrate degenerative changes without evidence of focal destructive osseous lesion.

IMPRESSION:

No discrete bladder mass identified or bladder wall hyperenhancement seen. Correlation with direct visualization and patient history is recommended. No evidence of metastatic disease identified within the abdomen or pelvis.

Diverticulosis without CT evidence of acute diverticulitis.

CT Scan report from OU Cancer Center that showed no sign of cancer or the tumor left behind.

I hope that all this has helped someone to understand my journey with cancer and taking the dog dewormer with Fenbendazole in it. I hope what I've done helps you or someone you know to fight to beat cancer. Just remember that for me the battle begins first in my mind with all the negative thoughts and emotions. THE MIND IS THE BATTLEFIELD. So stand strong. Ask for help if you can and do your research to find the answers you need to understand all you can do to help you. May the Spirit of the Universe be with you and the Miracle working power that it has to perform the unthinkable in our lives. If we can just lay aside our old ideas and beliefs to open the door to its awesome power, we can heal.

The cancer saved my life. If not for the cancer, I more than likely would not have known how bad my heart condition was and the true danger that was lurking within me. My primary care doctor sent me to see the cardiologist here in Ardmore to get it checked out. My first visit with him was on August 4, 2022. After him getting all my medical records from New Mexico, Oklahoma and reviewing them, he met with me to go over his findings. He came in and again I was told, "MR. BEST IT DOESN'T LOOK GOOD." He ordered me to have some procedures done to go into my heart to see if I had blockages and try to find out what was causing my condition. I returned and had the procedure done. I met with him at a later date to go over the results. He came in and said that I had a major blockage in the vein that feeds my heart with blood in a Y that appears to be 100% blocked and that it's called a WIDOW MAKER. I asked him why it's called that and he said when that type of blockage cause's a heart attack it makes your wife a widow. I laughed and said, "I don't have a wife!" He laughed. He then told me it was very serious and that he was going to send me to Oklahoma Heart Hospital South, in Oklahoma City, Oklahoma, to see the doctor to see if he could put in stents to help open up the blockages. I went in for the appointment and the doctor came in. My sister, Sudy, met me there to support me and be there to walk through all this with me. He started off with, "Mr. Best, it's pretty bad. The stent physician and I (the bypass physician) reviewed all of your records. We decided that we weren't willing to even attempt any type of procedure. We both feel your medical condition is too critical and that you wouldn't survive any surgery or that we would even be able to get you off the ventilator." I thought, "WOW, here I go again. Another DEATH SENTENCE STARING ME IN THE FACE!" Once again, my mind became the battlefield. I looked at him and asked, "Well, What NOW?" He then went on to tell me about the leading physician there named Doctor Tahirkheli (they call him Dr. T. for short) who sometimes works outside the box and attempts things that others wouldn't touch. If I was willing to talk to him, he would go visit with him about my case. I told him that I didn't have any other choice if I wanted to try to live. He left and told us to wait, we did. When he left the room, I looked at my sister and said, "Well, here we go again, another possible death sentence staring me in the face." He had asked me about the cancer and the dog dewormer I had taken. So I showed him all the documentation I had, with the photos and records I saved on my phone up to this point. After he looked at everything, he said that if anyone else had come in saying all this he would have thought that they were crazy, but since I had all this info with the reports, photos, recordings and everything I had to document all this, he had no choice but to believe me. After a long wait, four nurse's and four surgeons, along with Dr. T. came into the room. He introduced himself with all the others and began to tell me what they decided would be the best possible plan to help me. He said, "However, it is a very dangerous procedure and you might not survive." I asked him what he thought my chance was and he said, "I can't tell you that Mr. Best.

That's between you and GOD!" I immediately felt a sense of comfort and felt it's all in GOD'S hands! I agreed to let them do whatever they thought was to be done. He then asked me about the cancer. The other doctor told him about it and the dog dewormer. I showed him what I had on my phone and he asked about the pathologist report and if I had a PET Scan. I found all that on the phone and showed it to them. He looked at me and said, "MR. BEST YOU ARE A MIRACLE." He looked at the others in the room and said that they would have to start some research into this. I told them about Joe Tippen from Edmond, Oklahoma, located just North of where we were, and a little about his story of how he found out about the use of Fenbendazole. He shook my hand and they all left and told me the nurse would be back to set up the appointment to come in for the surgery. When they all left Sudy looked at me and said, "The moment Dr. T. mentioned God, your whole face lit up, and your voice changed." The reason I believe this happened is because when he said it was up to me and God, the very same thought I had earlier come to mind, "I GOT THIS EARNEST, JUST HAVE FAITH."

At this point there is something I would like to tell you, first I want to say that again I'm not a preacher. I'm not trying to get you to believe anything. I'm only trying to share my life story with you all and maybe give you some HOPE that maybe, just maybe, you too can find a miracle that can save your life as well. You see, from my earliest childhood memories I have been around and heard about God. I was a young child about three or four years old when my Father and Mother divorced. My father (Lawrence Best) was in the military in Columbia, South Carolina when he met my mother and they married. She was from a small town in Eastern South Carolina called Andrews. My Father left the military and we moved to Andrews, South Carolina. We were living there when they divorced. My Father took me when he left and brought me to Schulter, Oklahoma. It was a small village in between Okmulgee and Henryetta, Oklahoma, where his mother and father lived. He brought me there to live with them while he went out, coast to coast, as a truck driver. His sister, Verla Terry, lived next door to his parents with her Son and Husband. My Dad's Mom and Sister were very religious people, members of an old school Church of Christ. They, along with myself, attended every Sunday, Sunday night and Wednesday night without fail. These were my first memories of church and hearing about God. My Dad would come in off the road, after being gone for weeks at a time, and I remember being so excited to see him. He was a drinker and when he came in he would get all dressed up and go out on the town, sometimes for a few days before he would return. But he always found a few hours or a day that he would spend with me. He had a girlfriend and would go see her to spend time with her and her kids. I didn't understand all this back then. Sometimes I would get upset because he wouldn't take me with him. I started first grade there in Schulter. Years went by and Grandma was getting old. Grandma became diabetic and had to have her lower leg amputated. She was having a lot of health problems and told my Dad she was getting where it was too much for her to try to take care of me. He married his girlfriend and I went to live with them. I was about nine or ten by this time. He had a new job as a mechanic and came off driving the trucks for a while. I never went to church much back then. It was a totally different family environment and rules. They liked to drink and go out to parties, leaving us home to have Danny, the oldest stepbrother, babysit us. We ran wild and free getting into all kinds of mischief and trouble. We moved around a lot to different towns. My Dad would find better paying jobs and we would move to wherever the job was. We finally settled down in a small town in central Oklahoma called Wetumka. I was about 13 years old by then and started getting into a lot of trouble. I wouldn't mind my Stepmom and she had enough of me misbehaving. Dad was tired of my behavior as well, so they turned me over to the courts and placed me in foster care. I was sent to different foster homes and ended up in a place called Taft, a Juvenile home for kids in Muskogee, Oklahoma, (which now is a men's prison). A school teacher from Wetumka and her husband went to the courts and got me transferred from Taft to the Methodist Boys Ranch in Gore Oklahoma, on Lake Tenkiller. We attended church in Gore every Sunday and Sunday night. I was being taught of a different type of God by the Methodists than I had been taught about in the Church of Christ. I had been to several different types of church in foster care and all of them had different ideas and beliefs about God, Jesus and the Holy Spirit. By this time, I was really confused and didn't understand what to believe about it all. Some said God was Hell Fire and Damnation keeping a book with all my wrongs in it and I would go to hell for my wrongs. Today I think that was them trying to put the FEAR OF GOD in me to try to get me to behave! When I was about 15 my Mother came to Oklahoma from South Carolina to spend time with me. She came to visit me every weekend at the Boys Ranch. Her counselor in South Carolina told her it would be good for her to try to have a relationship with me. She had a drinking problem and was trying to get sober to straighten out her life. My Dad's Mom passed away from her diabetes. My Dad's sister and my Mom had always liked each other so she went to stay with her for a while. My Aunt Verla, my Dad's sister, and Grandpa would bring Mom up to the Boys Ranch every weekend to visit. My Dad and Stepmom had divorced. Dad and my Mom came to visit me and met with my counselor at the Ranch. My Mom decided to go back to South Carolina to get my brother James, who we call Peanut, and move back to Oklahoma. Mom and her Boyfriend had gone somewhere one night and got into an argument about something. She got out of the car and was walking along the side of the road when she got run over and died. My Dad came to the Ranch and told me what happened and they let me pack all my stuff and go home with him to go to South Carolina for her funeral. I was hurt and didn't understand why all this could happen. I blamed God for it all, everything, all the stuff I had been through, the sexual abuse by my cousin, the abandonments, the death of Grandma, just everything and I shut the door to God. I wanted nothing to do with any of the Gods I had been told about! They said God loves me. Well, if this is LOVE, then I don't want any part of it! This was the core of my belief about

God. I'm done! My Dad and I went to South Carolina for my Mom's funeral and returned to Wetumka. I stayed with him. He bought a house and we lived there together for a while. I started back to school and all went well for a while. Then he and my stepmom got back together. The school teacher and her family wanted me to come live with them, so I did. They had three sons and they were a lot different than any family I had previously lived with. They didn't drink or party and they went to a Methodist Church there in Wetumka. The husband was the Postmaster at the post office and she was the Choir and Chorus Teacher at the High School. Their sons were all good young men and they had a very nice home with a pool in the backyard. By this time, I was about 17 and a Junior in High School. They tried to help get me straightened out and had taken me to see Norman Vincent Peale at a Power of Positive Thinking Conference. Good stuff it was. I read some books they gave me by Zig Ziglar as well, all which helped me.

I discovered alcohol by this time. I took my first drink at the show in Wetumka one Saturday night when I was 15 and still living with my Dad. I walked into the restroom and a friend was in there and had a bottle, a half pint of Arriba wine. He asked me if I wanted a drink and I asked him what it was. He said, "Arriba wine and it's good." So I had a drink. It didn't take too much and we knocked out the half pint. He asked me if I had any money so he could go get us another bottle. I gave him what I had and he left to get us another one. After he left, I used the restroom and walked over to the sink to wash my hands. As I looked up at myself in the mirror, the MAGIC HAPPENED! I felt a warmness come up in my belly and as I looked at myself, my feelings and thinking began to change. All the grief from my Mothers passing went away. All the fears left, the shame and guilt left, the hate went away. I was better looking, so I thought. I remember looking into my eyes and saying out loud to myself, "I LIKE THIS!" The birth of my OBSESSION to use alcohol to change the way I think and feel was born in me that night! I fell in love with the effect that alcohol gave me that night. I'm going to try to explain something that happened to me when I was a child. When I told my Grandmother about the sexual abuse that was done to me back in Schulter when I still lived with her I was about eight or nine. I really don't remember the exact age, but I remember what happened. When I told her what was going on, she confronted my cousin about it. He denied it and convinced her I was lying. I got a whooping for lying. I wasn't telling any lies. I was scared and afraid. I felt that I was all alone. As I was outside playing with my Tonka Truck something happened in my mind, thoughts began to come. It was like a voice talking to me in my mind, telling me it's going to be okay Earnest. I have since learned that this was the birth of my EGO coming alive to comfort me. That voice became the guiding force of my life, my HIGHER POWER if you will. Everything I ever did I did because that voice told me it was the thing to do. That very same voice is the one that told me that night looking at myself in the mirror at the show, after feeling the effects of the alcohol I drank, "I LIKE THIS." I call it a voice, some people call it thoughts, to me it's the same. A very powerful thing. Since I had been around so many different Christian people, I knew what was right and wrong. But at times, I would do the very thing I knew was wrong and justify it or blame somebody else for my actions. People would sometimes ask me, "Earnest, why do you do the things you do?" and I couldn't answer them. I could only say two things, one was "I don't know" or "because I was drunk or high." Today the answer is because the thoughts crossed my mind and I had no defense against them. I can reflect back on my life today and see where there have always been two types of thoughts or voices that I can remember, one telling me to do what was right, the other was telling me to do what wasn't right, a selfish self-centered thought. This is the place I like to call the "BATTLEFIELD OF THE MIND." I know you all must think I'm crazy. Well, I too used to think the same thing, but once I got into recovery I heard another man tell his story about his own struggle with this type of insane thinking. I heard how he was able to resolve this issue. I then was able to talk about my insanity and find help to recover. For example, when I was told I had cancer, the negative thoughts began to come into my mind from somewhere. I have come to believe that they must come from a Spiritual Realm beyond our conscious capabilities to control with our Willpower. Lord knows I have told myself I'm not going to think things only to end up thinking the very thing I told myself I wasn't going to think about anymore, I have told myself I wasn't going to do certain things that I knew I shouldn't do, or that I didn't want to do anymore, only to do the very thing those thoughts had told me I wasn't going to do. Then I would have all these negative emotions, guilt and shame from my actions. As I look back, I can say that for a long time this struggle has been in my mind and a conflict within myself. I can only speak for myself, but I believe the struggle between RIGHT AND WRONG is as old as man itself. I believe this is called FREE WILL, and mine seemed to be broken.

When I took that first drink of wine it changed my thoughts and feelings. I felt relief from a lot of negative emotions. Like taking an aspirin for a headache, and I liked the effect it gave so it became my ASPIRIN for a good portion of the rest of my life. I never had anyone tell me about this BATTLE that goes on in some of us or how to deal with it until I got into recovery.

Some people call this voice or type of thinking the EGO, some call it EVIL SPIRITS, DEMONS, SELF and the list could go on. But whatever it is, it's a cunning, powerful and baffling thing to go through without help. When I got into recovery, they told me I was going to have to admit I was POWERLESS over the OBSESSION to drink or use in order to change the way I feel or think. Well after many attempts to stop and change I failed repeatedly.

As an example of how these thoughts just entered my mind, I will give you this example. The day they told me I was going to die from bladder cancer in six months to a year, and there wasn't anything that they could do to help me, the thoughts that came after being clean and sober for over ten years was, "WHAT THE HELL EARNEST, JUST GET YOU A HALF GALLON OF

CROWN ROYAL, A SACK OF DOPE, A PRETTY GIRL AND GO OUT IN A BLAZE OF GLORY!" Where on earth did those thoughts come from after all the things alcohol and drugs had done to me in my life, all the trouble I had gotten myself into, how many times I had relapsed before thinking it would be different, and all the misery I had put myself through. The family and friends I had hurt. I thank God I had been in recovery and had been able to repair the Spiritual Malady by asking God to put a hedge of protection around my thoughts and emotions. Asking Him to be there to intervene and protect my mind from such thoughts as those. Since I have worked through the resentments I had with God and all the prejudice I acquired towards Him, along with the fear of the unknown, I have been able to have a relationship with Him. This required letting go of all my old ideas about the Gods of religion I had been exposed to in my youth. I'm so thankful that He was there in my mind to put the thoughts in me to not act on those negative thoughts. But instead to give myself to research so maybe I could help find a possible treatment for this type of cancer to help save other people's lives. He gave me the desire to do this. I sought out some place to work with me, but found no one who was even willing to accept me because of the type of cancer I had. I want to share one more story with you that opened my eyes and heart to the fact that the Spirit of the Universe can live within us, putting thoughts and desires in our mind to help us. I had been in recovery for a few years back in the early 1990's and one day I realized that the OBSESSION to drink and use drugs had been removed. I hadn't thought about it in a long time. I prayed to God to help me have more faith and do His will and one day I had what's called a SPIRITUAL EXPERIENCE.

I had an old 1967 Chevy pickup. I rebuilt the engine, a high performance 396, and I was living in the Broadway House, a halfway house for recovering alcoholics and addicts in Ardmore, Oklahoma. This was in the early 1990's. I had been in and out of recovery and couldn't seem to get the recovery part to stick. I would get clean and sober, then relapse over and over. I first went to treatment in December of 1981 and found out that I was an alcoholic and drug addict. I decided to start the new engine and take it out for a test drive to break it in a little. I headed out of town on the access road alongside I-35. As I drove along, I spotted out of the corner of my eye, a lady standing up in the edge of the trees in a green dress. A thought crossed my mind, "STOP AND PICK HER UP." I kept driving, then the same thought came again, "STOP

AND PICK HER UP." It seemed a little louder this time, but I kept driving. Then it seemed to get overwhelming, this time "STOP AND PICK HER UP!!!!" It was accompanied with the hair standing up on my arms, with neck and goose bumps all over my body! I didn't know what was happening. I had never in my life experienced this before. So I stopped and backed up to where she was. She came out of the trees, walked up to the passenger side of my pickup and I said, "DO YOU NEED A RIDE?" She said she really needed something to drink. I had stopped and bought a coke before leaving town and I offered it to her. She took it and began to drink. It was in mid-August and it was hot. She was an older Black lady, really dark skinned and she had put mud all over her face. I assumed it was to try to protect her from the sun. She had a pillowcase with something in it. I asked her, "Do you need a ride somewhere?" She said, "Yes sir, maybe to the next truck stop." I thought for a second. Since at that time we didn't have any truck stops in Ardmore I could take her down the Interstate to the next town called Marietta, just south of Ardmore, about 18 to 20 miles. That trip would be good to get out on the Highway to break in my new engine, so I told her, "SURE, GET IN." She did. When she got in and placed the pillow case in the seat, I noticed it had a Bible in it and what appeared to be some clothes. I drove back through town to get to the on ramp for I-35. I stopped at a red light and as I looked across the street there was a Burger King. The thought crossed my mind to ask her if she was hungry, she said, "Yes sir." So I pulled in up to the drive through and told her to order whatever she wanted. She said for me to get her whatever I wanted her to have. I responded with "How long has it been since you ate?" She said, "Oh about three or four days now." I said, "WOW." I ordered a Double Whopper with cheese, fries and asked her if she wanted a drink or a malt. She said, "A chocolate malt sounds good." I ordered it for her. We got her order and I headed out to the on ramp and up on the Interstate South to Marietta. She began to pray over her meal so I stayed silent and just listened. She then began to drink her malt and eat her meal as I drove along. We didn't say much. She was really enjoying her food and drink. After she finished it all she said, "Thank You May God Bless You." I said, "Thank You." She then asked me if I went to church anywhere and I told her about being really confused with all of the different types of religions. I told her I had been involved with many different religions and wasn't at that time going to any church. I let her know I was in a 12 step program, trying to change my life and figure out what I should do. Then I asked her where she was headed and she said she was going south for the winter. I asked her where she was from and she said she had no home. I asked her how long she had been out here hitchhiking, and she said, "Oh about 11 or 12 years, I guess." I introduced myself and told her my name and she said her name was "Mary." I asked her well, what are you doing out here along the highway? She said she was saving souls for the Lord. The next thought that came was, "OH MY GOSH, this lady is crazy. She must have escaped from the NUT HOUSE!" She began to talk about Jesus, the Holy Spirit and about God. I just listened as she talked. I heard all this before, then she began to talk about the Holy Spirit, that Jesus told the followers about and how He would come and live in them after He left and God would send Him if they just believed. By this time, we were almost to the exit to get off for the truck stop. As I entered the off ramp and got close to the stop sign, she saw two people sitting under the bridge in the shade and said for me to let her off there. She said God wanted her to talk to them. As I pulled up to where the couple was sitting I asked her how she knew that God wanted her to talk to them? She said, "HE JUST TOLD ME." As I stopped I looked at her and said, "I DIDN'T HEAR HIM SAY ANYTHING!" She opened the door, stepped out, turned, looked me straight in the eyes and said, "BABY, YOU HAVE TO LEARN TO LISTEN TO THAT STILL SMALL VOICE IN YOUR MIND THAT'S THE SPIRIT OF GOD." I had the thought to give her the change left over from buying her the meal. I tried to give it to her and she wouldn't take it. She said she didn't need it because she had the faith to believe that God would provide for her needs. She had no idea about the prayers I had been praying, asking God to help me have more faith in Him and about the Mental battle I had prior to picking her up. She knew none of this, as she stared me in the eyes I asked her this, "HOW CAN YOU BELIEVE THAT GOD WILL PROVIDE YOUR NEEDS AND BELIEVE ALL THAT?" She then said what has changed my life forever, "HE TOLD YOU TO PICK ME UP AND FEED ME!" As I looked her in the eyes I felt the presence of an overwhelming love. I had goose bumps all over my body and I don't even know how to describe the feelings I had at that moment. It was like I was looking into the eyes of God's Spirit that was living in her. She said, "MAY GOD BLESS YOU." She shut the door and walked over to the couple. I drove off and entered the on ramp to return home and then it hit me. The thoughts began to flow through my mind like never before. It was so bad I had to pull over on the on ramp and stop. The tears flowed from deep inside of me and the thought came as plain as someone speaking to me, "SEE EARNEST I HAVE BEEN RIGHT HERE YOUR WHOLE LIFE." I saw for the first time that the still small voice that was telling me to pick her up must have been the Spirit of God living in me and trying to tell me what He wanted me to do. I had no idea at that time it was Him. I had never asked God before to reveal Himself to me and give me a sign to let me know He was real. Through this experience I believe He did just that.

From that day forward my life began to change and I had a lot of crazy thoughts. I told myself I must be crazy, I didn't want to tell anyone about all this because of my fear of what they might think. All kinds of negative things trying to steal away the very thing that was trying to give me faith. You see all my life I made fun of people who would say they heard from God or say God had told them something. I just had a lot of old ideas and beliefs from what I had been taught growing up. But now, how could I ever deny what had just happened? I couldn't and I haven't! It was on that day I realized a lot of things. One thing that came to mind was something I heard growing up that said, "Be kind to strangers because some have entertained Angels sent to help them on their Journey." In my heart I believe that this old Black lady, hitchhiking down the interstate with mud all over her face, was possibly an Angel sent to answer my prayers. I had been praying that God would show me He was real and His Spirit was alive and living in my mind, trying to give me directions. But because I have always been so into SELF AND EGO DRIVEN THOUGHTS I couldn't hear Him. That's the place I call the BATTLEFIELD. When thoughts are telling me to do one thing and another set of thoughts is telling me to do the next right thing, the BATTLE begins. And without help from the Spirit of the Universe, which I call GOD, I lose the Battle! There is absolutely no way that lady could have known anything about the mental battle I had before I picked her up, or the prayers I had been praying! Just like the veterinarian was put into Joe Tippens life to give him directions to take the dog dewormer to save his life. Joe Tippen was put in my life to tell me about the dog dewormer. All those people who text me telling me about the dog dewormer that has saved my life. The BATTLEFIELD OF THE MIND, a book by Joyce Myers, I got while I was in prison helped open my mind to this battle ground of our thoughts, the 12 step program that was given to Bill W. and Dr. Bob, along with 100 others who put it all together in a book called, Alcoholics Anonymous, that has saved many millions and helped them have a Spiritual Awakening that has changed their lives and helped them straighten out their own Spiritual Malady's.

I hope I haven't lost your interest in all this. I just felt a need to try and explain why I say so much about the mental battle we have within ourselves. I know not all of you may even be able to relate. But those of you who can, you know what I say is true.

So back to the heart surgery. I returned home to Ardmore to wait for the first attempted surgery to get through the blockage. It was a few weeks out so I had plenty of time. I was having a lot of chest pain, low oxygen levels, on oxygen 24/7, having bad muscle cramps when I would try to walk or do anything, so I just had to take it easy.

They set up my appointment for the surgery on May 23, 2023. By that time the chest pains had become worse and my heart rate would shoot up over 120 to 135 if I tried to do anything. Sometimes just laying around it would go crazy. I called Dr, T.'s office and they told me to come to Oklahoma City, OHH it's called, to the ER. So I did. I drove myself to Sudy's house in Tuttle and she drove me to the ER where I was admitted right away and taken to the Heart Ward. This was on May 21, 2023. On the morning of the 23rd they prepared me for the surgery. I was told again that it was a very high-risk surgery and they had me sign a bunch of release forms. They again told me it was a 50/50 chance that something could go wrong and I wouldn't survive. Right away my mind and thoughts took off crazy. I remember thinking that they have contacted Big Pharma and the CDC. Since I have been telling everyone about this miracle dog dewormer with FENBENDAZOLE treating my cancer, they might be fixin' to take me out!!! Then right behind that was the same thought as before, "HAVE FAITH EARNEST, I GOT THIS." I knew then that no matter what happened, it was going to be okay! So once again, and for the first time, I was standing in the face of possible death and I was at peace only by the Grace of the Spirit of the Universe! I signed all the papers and went over my last wishes with Sudy. I was ready to go. They took me to the surgery room and placed me on the table with a God awful bunch of lights, TV screens and it was cold as all get out. They covered me with warm blankets and began putting all kinds of stuff in me and on me. As I lay there looking up at the bright lights, I prayed and asked for forgiveness for anything I might have overlooked. I thanked God with gratefulness for the life He had given me and asked Him to at least be a greeter at the Gates of Heaven since I hadn't been no Saint. I thanked Him for being with me my whole life even though I didn't know He was even there. I heard Dr. T. tell them to prepare me to have an impeller pump put into my groin in case something unforeseen happens. I found out later that they are used to pump blood throughout the body if the heart stops. At least that's the way I understood the description. They placed the mask over my face and told me to count backwards from 100. They started injecting drugs in my arm. I barely remember getting to 90 and I was out. They told me the surgery was scheduled for five hours, but it was almost ten hours when I awoke in the Intensive Care Unit (ICU). When I came to myself the nurse was there, along with Sudy. I had stuff coming out of me everywhere! I had wires coming out of my jugular vein, a black and red one. The nurse told me to be very careful and don't unhook them or I would die. They went to my temporary pacemaker because during the surgery my heart stopped. I had a heart attack and died once already. Thank God Dr. T. had the last-minute thought to install the impeller pump that saved me until they could hook up the pacemaker. The next day they took me back into surgery and installed a permanent pacemaker that I have today. They say I'm 97% dependent on it to live. Once again, I thank

God for Dr. T. making the right decision to install the impeller pump. I was told that they are used to pump people's blood while they wait on a heart transplant. They removed it after surgery.

After a few days I went home in pretty bad shape. My body was beaten up and bruised. Coming off all of the drugs, Morphine, Fentanyl and who knows what else, and I couldn't hardly walk because of the impeller pump they had put in my groin area.

Dr. T. came in and went over the surgery with me. He said that the blockage was really bad. It was as hard as cement and he couldn't get a wire strong enough to go through it. He tried all sizes, but nothing would go. He tried balloons and a lot of stuff, but wasn't able to cross. Then my heart stopped so they had to get everything out and go to work to save my life and hook up the pacemaker. After he told me all this and left the room that day, I thought about all those crazy thoughts I had before the surgery. About them maybe going to take me out because of the dog dewormer and me spreading all that stuff around about it treating my cancer. They had the chance if they wanted to, it was the time and place and justifiable to do that day. Thank God that wasn't the case! I was sent home with a home pacemaker monitor that records and sends out the result to the pacemaker Doctor (I call him my Electrician) (Dr. T. is my plumber) I got a call from him and they wanted me to come in ASAP, saying that there was a problem with the pacemaker. I had noticed my heart rate was going crazy and having chest pains really bad, so I left out and went to Oklahoma City. When I got to his office, they checked my pacemaker again and took me to a room and admitted me. I asked them what was going on and they said one of the wire's had come out of my heart and it wasn't working right. They were going to have to go back in and do the surgery again to put it back into my heart. The wires have a corkscrew on the ends that screw into the heart and the heart grows around it over time. I didn't follow their instructions well and I must have put my arms up over my head while I slept which pulled it out. Once again, my life was saved. Thank God Again!

After a day in the hospital, I came back home to Ardmore to rest and heal up for a while before going back to see Dr. T. to try the blockage surgery again. I returned in January 2024. I was admitted and had a blood test prior to surgery. They came into the room and said I had lost all my blood and that my blood count was down to 6.2. They said I was losing a lot of blood somewhere and they advised me that they couldn't do the surgery until they found out what was going on. They told me that when our blood count falls below 7, it is critical and that I must have blood transfusions ASAP. Dr. T. came in and ordered a bunch of different doctors to come check me out. They needed to find out where I was bleeding. I was shocked as I had seen no blood loss coming from anywhere. I was baffled. They asked me about my stools and what color it was. I told them it had been black for a while. I thought it was black because of the Folgers instant coffee I drank or the meds they had me on. They said, "No Mr. Best, coffee won't do that, but black stools mean internal bleeding somewhere." I DIDN'T KNOW THAT! They stopped all my meds, blood thinners and aspirin. They started giving me blood transfusions, a total of three units, and a unit of Iron as well. That brought my blood count up to 8.1. They started getting me ready to have an Upper GI and a colonoscopy to try to locate the bleeding. After a day to get me ready for the procedure, they came in, knocked me out again and found several things that were bleeding. They stopped it all. Thank God, again!!

Dr. T. came in and said that he wanted to get me off the Eliquis blood thinner and that they had a new type of help for me called a Watchman Device. He explained that due to the AFib and strokes they had me on it. He explained that we have a small pocket in our hearts that collects blood and forms blood clots. The blood thinners cause them to come out and cause us to have a stroke. This device is placed in the opening to that pocket to seal off the clots from coming out to cause a stroke. I don't know how it helps AFib, but I told him sure if he thought I should, then let's do it. They scheduled an appointment. I returned and had the surgery done to install it. Here another miracle happened. In order to install the Watchman, they have to go through the right chamber of the heart to make an incision into the left chamber going into it to get to the pocket to install it. It works like a small parachute that opens up and over a few weeks the heart grows around it and seals it off. But when they made the incision between the chambers, it relieved the pressure and since they put it in I have had no chest pains or discomfort. I'm completely off all the oxygen. My heart and overall health has dramatically improved.

There was another surgery that I overlooked to try to get through the blockages that I had before the bleeding problem. It was a failure as well due to all the other surgeries and radiation exposure. When they were attempting the procedure I became overdosed with radiation. We are only allowed to have so much exposure then they have to stop. After several hours, Dr. T. had been able to finally get a wire through one side of the blockage, but wasn't able to open it up due to the radiation exposure. I was told that they noticed my heart was building its own bypass around both sides of the blockages using other veins. Over time it may complete them and I would be okay. So, it's all in God's Hands at this time, Many Miracles have happened and are still happening!

I returned to see Dr. T. after the Watchman Device was installed for a follow up. He said that they are still doing research into the reason all my heart problems improved after the incision between the chambers. He said the Watchman has no effect on anything other than to block the pocket, but the incision has done something. Since everything has changed. I'm not having any problems and doing so much better, he doesn't want to attempt it again unless I start having chest pains or problems.

Today everything is good. I feel great. No chest pains, no oxygen problems, no irregular heartbeat, no signs of any cancer. My health has improved beyond reason and I can only say that to me this is truly MIRACULOUS and a MIRACLE from the Spirit of the

Universe, GOD, JESUS, HOLY SPIRIT, DIVINE, or whatever your faith or belief is.

He has put many people in my life and worked through them to save me from all this. This story started off about my journey with cancer and the death sentence I was given, with no possible treatments or anything that could be done for me. He put people in my life to tell me what to do to save my life, to take a DOG DEWORMER of all things to kill it! He put all the other doctors in my life that found the other problems I had so they could save my life and they did. The blockages, the bleeding out, the impeller pump, the Watchman Device, He has truly worked through so many people to save me for some reason. I believe it is to show others about His awesome MIRACLE working powers and how much He can and will do if we just BELIEVE! You see, I once had resentments, fears and a rebellion towards Him. I truly had a SPIRITUAL MALADY and refused to form a relationship with Him. I got angry anytime anyone would talk about GOD, JESUS, or the HOLY SPIRIT. It brought out my rebellion, the anger, the prejudice, old ideas from childhood religions and all that stuff.

It's been a long hard road since December of 1981, when I was sent to treatment for Alcoholism and Drugs.

This thing in me has fought it all the way. That voice I talk about in my mind or the thoughts that come from somewhere that resist surrendering to anything other than itself. They told me that drinking and drugging was just a symptom of the problem, that I drank and did drugs to change the way I feel and think. That I was EGO driven, full of selfishness and self-centered to the extreme. That I had formed an OBSESSION with alcohol and drugs and that I was powerless over that OBSESSION. I refused to believe that and fought it tooth and nail. I can't tell you how many times I tried to CONTROL my thoughts and actions telling myself, "I'M DONE I'M NOT DRINKING NO MORE," only to last a few days or weeks then the thoughts would come again and tell me I can control it this time. Just drink a beer or just have a couple, only to wake up drunk again or in jail for something I had done. They told me I had an Alcoholic Mind. They said my thinking that PRECEDES a relapse into drinking is the CRUX of my problem. They said that when the thoughts come into my mind from somewhere I have no effective mental defense against them. This made me angry! I wasn't going to admit I was powerless over my ability to control my thoughts. In my mind the only thing I thought I was powerless over was the effects that the alcohol produced. People used to tell me, "EARNEST

YOU'RE A PRETTY GOOD OLE BOY TILL YOU START DRINKING," so I thought that alcohol was the problem. I could see that once I started to drink, I couldn't stop until I was drunk or passed out or ended up in jail for fighting, outrunning the police or something that would stop me for a time. They told me my life was UNMANAGEABLE. I just wouldn't believe that only when I was drunk was it unmanageable because of the effects of alcohol. They told me I had a thinking problem, but oh no, I don't think I have a thinking problem! Well, it has taken me many years to reach that place that I know in my Heart of Hearts that my thinking is where my problem is. After many relapse's, jails, a 15 year prison sentence for drugs (that I served five and one half years on), countless damaged relationships, loss of good jobs, loss of everything I owned, living on the streets homeless, attempted suicides, countless trips to mental institutions, treatment centers for alcoholism and drugs, and the list goes on. They told me that a lack of POWER was my Dilemma, and that I was going to have to find a power which would solve my problem! I came back to the 12 step program in September of 1999, to try it again, for the fourth or fifth time. I haven't had any form of alcohol for nearly 25 years in September. The OBSESSION with alcohol has been removed. I haven't had the thought to drink but a few times since then, like the day they told me I was going to die from this cancer. Thank God I found a relationship with a power greater than myself that was right there to put the next thoughts in my mind to do something different other than drink! "MY MIND IS THE BATTLEFIELD" I have finally come to accept and believe based on the FACTS OF LIFE that I indeed have a thinking problem. I am powerless over where thoughts come from and that in a moment of temptation, I have no defense against the thought. I must depend on a power outside myself that can and will intervene to save me and put the next right thought in my mind. I have tried every imaginable thing I can come up with to defend my mind against this BATTLE when it occurs, and have failed every time sooner or later. In regard to my Alcohol problem it truly has been removed and the obsession is gone. Now about the drugs, I never was able to admit I had a drug problem or that I was an addict because in my sick mind I thought an addict was someone who used a needle, not prescription drugs, or pot, or speed, or Quaaludes, white crosses, bird eggs or any other form of speed. When I found the caffeine pills (white crosses) you could order from Hustler Magazine, Bird Eggs and the like I thought I found the cure to getting drunk. They would allow me to get wired up and drink more and I liked that new magical fix. No more blackouts, just drink and drink. Then came snorting Cocaine, PCP speed, meth and whatever else came my way, but no needles. I wasn't going to be a drug addict so I thought! Well, that's all changed. In April of 2012, I got busted for endeavoring to manufacture meth. I plead guilty and was facing a 20 to Life sentence. The Judge only gave me 15 years and I went to prison for five and one half years. During the time I started using meth, the desire to drink never came. I never had a drink of any alcohol all that time. A true MIRACLE! When I was in the County Jail waiting to pull a chain they called it (THAT'S WHEN YOU GO TO PRISON). I had a lot of time to get honest and take a good long honest look at my life and see that, yes, they are right. MY BEST THINKING BROUGHT ME HERE, HEADED TO PRISON FOR 15 YEARS. All the things I learned and experienced in the past 31 years at that time started to come back to me, running through my mind every day. The old lady hitchhiker and what she had done to me, all the things that I had read, the things people told me. It was endless. I remembered the hitchhiker patting that Bible and telling me all of my answers were in there. I found a Bible in jail and started to read and study it everyday. I had never done that. I would just go to church and listen to whoever was teaching, who was reading His Book tell me what he thought it meant. My mind had fought reading that book with every fiber of my being!! I spent over a year in the County Jail waiting to go to prison. When I finally was taken to prison and sent to medium security in Eastern Oklahoma, called Jim Hamilton, they had a group of people from the free world who came once a week and held AA meetings that I attended every week. There was a man named Jerry Sickler from Mena, Arkansas, who had 30 plus years clean and sober who started the meetings, who today has passed away from COVID. When I heard him tell his story, he was the first man I had ever heard who had been through the same mental turmoil. He experienced the same things I had been going through for years. I asked him to be my sponsor and to please help me find the solution he had found. He agreed to help me! He asked me if I was convinced that my thinking was the problem? Was I driven by the bondage of Self and that my EGO was running my life. I honestly had no idea what the heck he was talking about. So he sent me on an educational journey to learn about the human Ego and the bondage it has over us alcoholics. He said I had missed something over the years and that we had to find out what it was. I knew how to get clean and sober. I just couldn't live with myself for long periods of time after I stopped using and would return to drink for relief from myself again and again. WHAT HAD I MISSED? After a few meetings with him, and studying about the Ego and self, I could see that, yes, I am convinced that they are the problem and not alcohol and drugs. Because of all the failures at trying to control my life, my thoughts and emotions to manage my life to the best of my ability, and failing every time, I couldn't deny the truth any longer! I had to be rigorously honest with myself and for the first time I admitted I was powerless, and my life was unmanageable by me alone. I had come to believe that it was going to take a power far greater than myself to help me! But how do I find this power since I'm angry at God? I have all these old ideas about Him. Prejudice, the fear of the unknown, rebellious, Ego driven and full of self that fights the very thought of surrendering to Him.

Jerry told me that I was suffering from a SPIRITUAL MALADY, and until I straighten that out, I probably would never make it! He said that I was going to have to come to believe in a power GREATER than myself that could restore me to sanity. He asked me if I believed in God and I tried to answer that question to the best of my ability. He asked me where I might find a concept of God and I answered, "THE BIBLE I GUESS." He then told me to write down all the things I would ask God, then read the New Testament and try to find my answers. So, I began the journey of research to try to find the answers. Boy did I ever find them all plus I found a lot of things I didn't have questions for. He asked me what stage of my disease of alcoholism I was in. I had no idea. I didn't even know it had different stages like cancer, so he sent me on the journey to find that out in the Big Book of Alcoholics Anonymous (AA). I found it and I told him I was in the last stage of my disease. I had grown to use sedatives and drugs to help me drink and function. I had become a TRUE ALCOHOLIC! Not an Alcoholic addict, but a TRUE, FULL BLOWN ALCOHOLIC!!!

We begin to work on the malady I had and walk through the resentments, fears, the old ideas, the childhood religions I had been exposed to, the blaming Him for things that wasn't His doing, a whole world of things that was blocking me off. The main thing was my thoughts and my mind telling me all kinds of stuff to block me from surrendering to Him and asking Him for help.

Once we walked through all this and I was at peace with turning all my crazy thoughts and Ego over to His care and asking Him to help me fight the BATTLE OF MY MIND everything began to change. I started every morning with asking Him to put a hedge of protection around my mind, my thoughts, and my emotions. I asked Him to be there if a thought of temptation was to enter my mind, to help me to stay clean, sober and of sound mind. To give me the next right thought and the ability to take action to overcome the temptation. I ask Him every night to do the same, to be there with me when I wake up to guard my thoughts because that's the hardest time to surrender to His will upon awakening. The thoughts were always there telling me to wait, to make coffee, or some off the wall reason to prolong and put off praying and connecting with Him.

I know today that my mind and ego can cause me great harm, but things are a lot better today. I hope that I have been able to give you HOPE and help someone else save their life. I hope that you too can begin to win the battle of your mind and fight the good fight to save your life. I have shared a lot with you and tried to relay the message of HOPE. I hope that the story about my cancer, my heart, my Alcoholism and drug addiction can help someone else to find a relationship with the Spirit of the Universe that can do many things in our lives if we just have faith and believe.

I would like to share some research I found during my journey. Over the years there has been a lot of research that explains exactly how Fenbendazole works at destroying parasitic worms as well as cancer cells. So far, there appears to be four different modes of action.

FIRST, around the nucleus of all living cells, there exists a protein-structured microtubule network. These microtubules are involved in cell division, the cell being able to adapt its shape to a changing environment, and the movement of compounds within the cell.

SECOND, Fenbendazole binds to tubulin, a structural protein of these microtubules. This creates a blockage in the tiny tubes and prevents the removal of waste products and the intake of nutrients. The uptake of GLUCOSE, THE SOLE ENERGY SOURCE OF THE PARASITIC WORMS, is shut down. Without an energy supply, the worms are either paralyzed and die, or they are expelled from the body.

CANCER CELLS also require GLUCOSE AS AN ENERGY SOURCE. By blocking the microtubular network of CANCER CELLS, Fenbendazole helps to shut down their energy supply and destroys them.

THIRD, Fenbendazole further increases the activity of the body's natural killer cells in the presence of P53 tumor suppressor genes.

FOURTH, Fenbendazole acts as a kinase inhibitor, which helps block the formation of new blood vessels necessary for tumors to survive.

These anticancer properties are not new. In 2002, while working for MD Anderson, Dr. Tapas Mukhopadhyay and his colleagues reported that mebendazole elicited a potent antitumor effect on human cancer cell lines both in vitro and in vivo.

In simple terms, Mebendazole (for all practical purposes the same drug as Fenbendazole) strongly and profoundly inhibited the growth of lung, breast, ovary, colon, and bone cancer cells in both tissue samples and in live animals. At the same time, it had no negative effects on normal cell growth.

This same study was supported by a grant from the National Cancer Institute. It makes you wonder why they would fund a study like this, get such amazing results, and then not have enough interest to do a follow-up study or further pursue a drug with such potential.

In 2009, researchers at John Hopkins evaluated various drugs for treatment of glioblastoma-the most common brain cancer in adults. It is very aggressive, with the average survival 11 to 15 months, and it is considered incurable.

They implanted the cancer cells into the brains of mice, which is the normal procedure in these types of studies. Before implanting the cells, however, these particular mice were treated with Fenbendazole. The brain cancer did not develop. It never grew.

Later in 2012, Dr. Mukhopadhyay and his colleagues, at Panjab University in India, published another study showing that Fenbendazole was a potent compound for inhibiting the growth of cancer cells without doing harm to or affecting the growth of normal cells.

And in 2018, Dr. Mukhopadhyay and his colleagues published yet another study highlighting Fenbendazole as a safe and inexpensive anthelmintic drug possessing "efficient antiproliferative activity" in human cells. (This basically means it inhibits the growth of cancer cells).

Fenbendazole is considered an animal product. It was never approved for human use. It's sold without a prescription. Its patent has expired so anyone can make it generically. This is why no individual or company wants to promote it or recommend it for use in humans.

To get Fenbendazole approved for humans could cost hundreds of millions of dollars. No one is willing to spend that kind of money without patent protection and the ability to recoup their money.

I found this article "A CURE FOR CANCER…HIDDEN IN PLAIN SITE" this is just a small part of the article I wanted to share, please look it up and read it for yourself.

I have shared a lot about my life and the journey with you. Again, I want to say that I'm no doctor, preacher, or salesman of anyone's products. I'm trying to relay a message of HOPE to all who read these pages and are looking for a possible way to live. To find a way to stop this deadly disease of cancer from taking their life, to maybe find a miracle along their journey.

If you are reading this book to find help for yourself or if you are a family member who is trying to help a loved one find a possible treatment, I want to say that it's very important to not stop this protocol once you find recovery. It is very important that we all continue the regimen, even if the cancer improves, the test and scans all come back NED, or if you just wish to stay cancer free. I have shared with a few that have started the protocol, found amazing results, became cancer free, then stopped the protocol. They went back to the old way of life, were doing the same things as before and the cancer came back. Some have died because the cancer is sometimes a silent killer. We don't know it is present until it has spread throughout the body and taken over to the point of no return, causing them to lose the battle.

In my research I found that cancer remains the leading health concern for most people, with over 1.9 million new diagnoses and an estimated 600,000 deaths expected in the United States this year alone. Because of numbers like that is why I wanted to put this message in a book to try to share my journey that has, so far, saved my life. Maybe, just maybe, it will help to save others with this possible good news. Everything I say and write here is my own journey and story of what I have done as a cancer survivor, my own research and findings.

I have many friends who have seen what Fenbendazole has done for me and many others so far and have started taking it as a preventive measure to try to avoid ever getting cancer. They ask me for advice on what they should do. Since I still use Fenbendazole to prevent the cancer from coming back, I tell them to do what I do now. Here is what I tell them to do and it is only my advice to them and whomever else may wish to know. I tell them to start a protocol for at least one month that consists of 222 mgs of Fenbendazole a day, one 500mg turmeric/curcumin, and one 500 mgs magnesium once a day. Then stop taking the Fenbendazole, but to keep taking the turmeric and magnesium. Then every month take Fenbendazole 222 mgs for a week, along with the other stuff. I take a daily multivitamin as well. Be sure to take the Fenbendazole with a meal so it has the help of fatty foods or oils to help dissolve it in the stomach. I also found research that said periodic rest periods may be beneficial. So that's why I take it now once a month, for a week. So far, so good.

In my research I found that malignant cells seem unable to develop resistance to Fenbendazole with prolonged use, unlike traditional chemotherapy drugs. This enables long-term administration without loss of efficacy. A major way cancer cells develop chemoresistance is through P-glycoproteins-special pumps expelling anti-cancer drugs from the cell before they can exert effects. The research shows malignant cells do not identify Fenbendazole as a compound to eject via these pumps. So unlike other agents, Fenbendazole remains inside the cancer cells. By avoiding efflux by p-glycoproteins, Fenbendazole can retain its potency long-term.

During my research I asked Google, "HOW DOES FENBENDAZOLE WORK TO KILL CANCER? This is what I found.

Fenbendazole eliminates parasites by inhibiting the production of microtubules, which are structural components of cells that enable intracellular division. In other words, Fenbendazole stops mitosis by the same mechanism that kills parasites.

Fenbendazole attacks malignancies through several key pathways:

1. Triggering apoptosis (programmed cell death). It does this by arresting the cell cycle via microtubule disruption.

2. Restricting cancer cell glucose uptake. High glucose consumption fuels uncontrolled tumor growth. Fenbendazole appears to limit glucose and

this starves cells of division-enabling sugars.

3. Reactivating the tumor suppressor p53 gene. Fenbendazole restores p53 function, which is a strong tumor suppressor. Humans don't have much of this gene, but Fenbendazole helps to activate it.

Again, this is all research stuff that I have found about Fenbendazole and has helped me understand more about cancer and the effects of Fenbendazole. I wanted to share with you all to maybe help you to understand more. There is a great deal of additional research going on now than there was two years ago. Due to the overwhelming success of many people trying this drug. Many finding the same results and living cancer free. Once again, I want to say that all this information is just my personal thoughts and research into Fenbendazole. My cancer and everything else in this story is my own opinion.

In closing, I want to say that I wish you all the best possible outcomes and hope that you too may find the same results countless others, as well as myself, have found by taking the drug Fenbendazole. Many lives have been saved and some have passed away. I personally believe that if a person waits too long to attack this disease of cancer it spreads so fast and aggressively that once a certain point is reached cancer takes over and can't be stopped. When I found that the CDC recommends humans do a parasite cleanse every six months, I was shocked. I had never been told anything about that. When I found the story about Joe Tippen, read it and listened to his podcast, I was amazed again. Today, without ever having any kind of treatment to try to kill this cancer, no experimental drugs of any kind except Fenbendazole, Turmeric/Curcumin and Magnesium, I'm cancer free.

I'm another living example that it works. May God Bless you all and may you find the healing and miracles that await you. May you search deep within yourself and find what's causing your SPIRITUAL MALADY so you too might find what you seek and have a relationship with the Spirit of the Universe that can help you. Just remember THE MIND IS THE BATTLEFIELD!!!!

I truly believe what they told me years ago, "THAT WHEN THE SPIRITUAL MALADY IS OVERCOME, WE STRAIGHTEN OUT MENTALLY AND PHYSICALLY."

When we are told that we have CANCER, it's a life changing event, one that changes not only us but the ones closest to us, family, friends, co-workers who have to watch us go through this ordeal. Being given a possible DEATH SENTENCE with only a few months or days to live really is life changing. It's a very emotional time as well. As we reflect back over our lives and see the things we have neglected and been so caught up in LIFE that we didn't take time to stop and enjoy the people in our lives, or spend more time with them, as we question the God of our understanding as to why me? Like I said before, my mind became the BATTLEFIELD, lay down and die or stand up and fight!

I am so grateful that I have been given another chance at life and found a way to reach out and try to help as many others as I can with this book. To share my journey, so far, through all this with you all so that maybe you too can find healing and stand up against this disease and find HOPE.

Once again, I want to say that all this is my own journey using the dog dewormer with Fenbendazole in it that I truly believe saved my life. I'm so thankful for all of the people that was put in my life to give me the help I needed to fight this thing from the 12 step program, Joyce Myers book Battlefield Of The Mind, all the podcasts I have watched with Joel Osteen, Joe Tippen and his remarkable journey with cancer, along with the

Old Black lady hitchhiker, the research I have found everywhere about all this. But most importantly GOD, who has been the reason all these people have been put in my life to share with me to give me the course He wanted me to follow. I was able to take off the "Rose-colored glasses of rebellion," anger, fear, prejudice, religion, old ideas from childhood and judgement, the list could go on and on, and open the door with an open mind to seek out an understanding that felt right to me.

I had no idea that a small couple of minutes video in that convenient store would get posted on TikTok and go out all around the world to be shared and viewed over 50 million times. It still amazes me at the overwhelming impact it has had on so many people. Thank You for your time to read this book. Do your research. Learn all you can and FIGHT, FIGHT, FIGHT…

Sincerely yours,

—Earnest Best

A letter from one of my Heart Assistants who has witnessed my recovery with cancer and the drug Fenbendazole, along with all the heart problems and miracles. As well as other friends and acquaintences.

Earnest has a story that shines hope in the darkest areas for those experiencing cancer. While the method he describes is simple, his life and health is a testament to the amazing results he lays out in this book. Earnest's passion is in recovery - whether it be from cancer or substance abuse. His story speaks to the heart of all those struggling with the spiritual malady.

Many who find themselves separated from health, happiness and God will find in Earnest's journey a path not only to recovery of cancer, but a life of wholeness and inspiration.

Earnest continues to play a key role in my own life. As I see his method of treating cancer continue to work, my heart is filled with gratitude knowing he has many more years to be a part of my journey.

—S. Renfro

In his story Earnest Best relates an almost unbelievable tale. In fact, if I had not seen significant portions of his medical records and witnessed some of the events described, I probably wouldn't have believed it. This story of healing falls largely outside the scope of traditional medicine.

Even though Earnest is not a formally trained writer, he crafts a sincere heartfelt story that is both honest and deeply personal.

This book has the capacity to encourage, inspire, and comfort readers from all walks of life. The reader senses the vulnerability in the writing as Earnest wrestles intensely with his life, his demons, and a terminal diagnosis. This journey to healing and redemption is both powerful and profound. I am truly grateful that Mr. Best has chosen to share this story along with his experience, strength, and hope...

—Dr. Britt Morris
Vascular Surgeon, Retired

From the moment you begin reading this amazing life adventure story, you experience what it's like to be at the depths of addiction to the highs of God's life giving love. A most unusual route breaking from traditional medicine for incurable bladder cancer to a more traditional approach for his heart condition, along with another miracle occurring through faith, trust and surrender to "God, as he understands," that guided him to be delivered from mental anguish.

I'm a Urologist and my first connection to Earnest was in follow up to his initial surgery for bladder cancer when he returned to Oklahoma. But I really became a friend through my participation with my wife and her recovery in the 12 step program. So I can assure you that his story is real and his medical records are accurate.

As a reader you will be inspired by what a "life given to God" allows for growth, recovery and a joyous life to a capacity that you may never think possible.

—Hayden D. Henry, MD
Urologist

I met Earnest Best at the 12 step program, we both attended. Earnest's story is amazing and shows that God can use different ways to heal. At our meetings Ernest always says something that inspires me. What he shared one day gave me the courage to restore my relationship with my sister that had been "destroyed" by my behavior. I love Ernest. His story will inspire those who read it.

—**Lisa Henry**

When Mr. Best first reached out to us, his heartfelt conviction and deep spiritual commitment to sharing his journey left a lasting impression. We're truly honored to have played a part in bringing this extraordinary story to light—a story we believe has the power to profoundly change the lives of all who read it.

—Maurice and Rita Johnson
Self Publish Me

Contact the author:

I truly enjoy connecting with readers and sharing my journey. If you'd like to discuss a speaking engagement, book signing, or another event, please email me at: ernieleebest63@gmail.com

www.ingramcontent.com/pod-product-compliance
Lightning Source LLC
Chambersburg PA
CBHW050655160426
43194CB00010B/1947